Illustrated Christmas Poetry

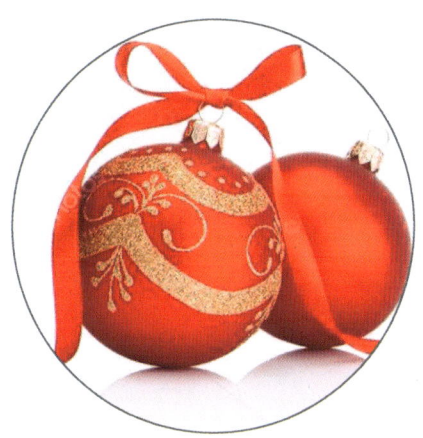

This book of verses from traditional and classic poems belongs to:

_____

The 12 Days of Christmas

On the first day of Christmas

my true love sent to me

A partridge in a pear tree.

On the second day of Christmas

my true love sent to me

Two turtle doves,

And a partridge in a pear tree.

Traditional song

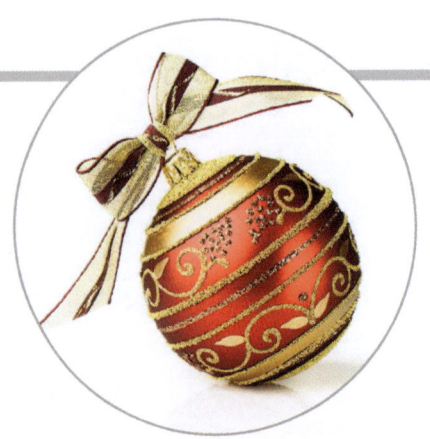

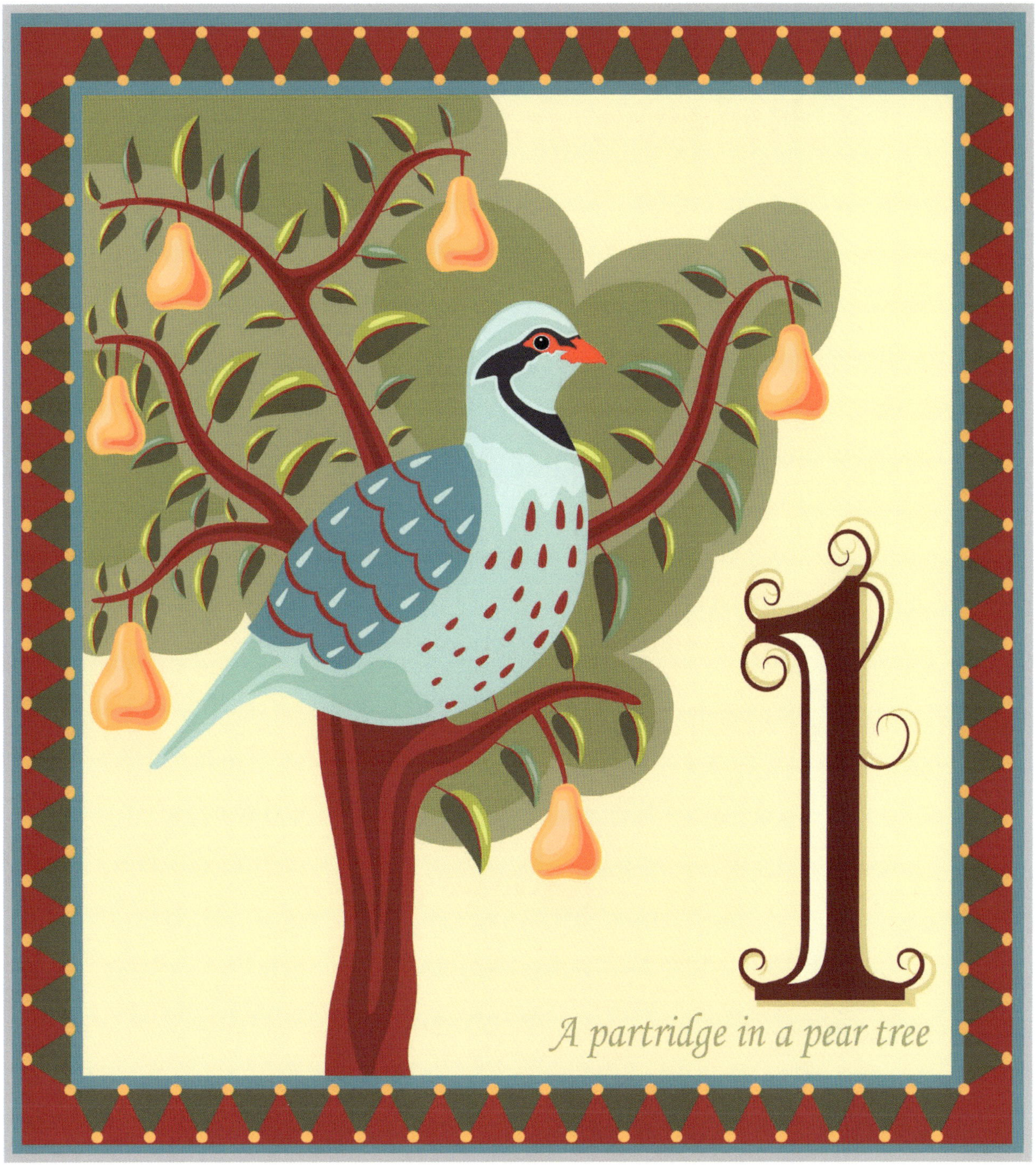

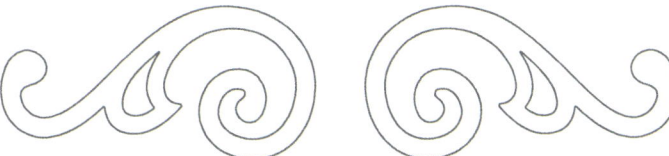

A partridge in a pear tree

1

Christmas is Coming

Christmas is coming,

    the goose is getting fat.

Please do put a penny

    in the old man's hat.

If you haven't got a penny,

    a ha'penny will do.

If you haven't got a ha'penny,

    then God bless you!

Traditional rhyme

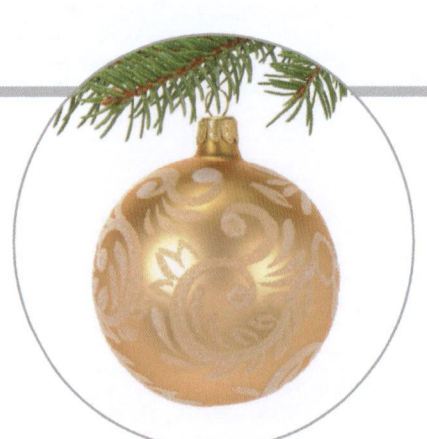

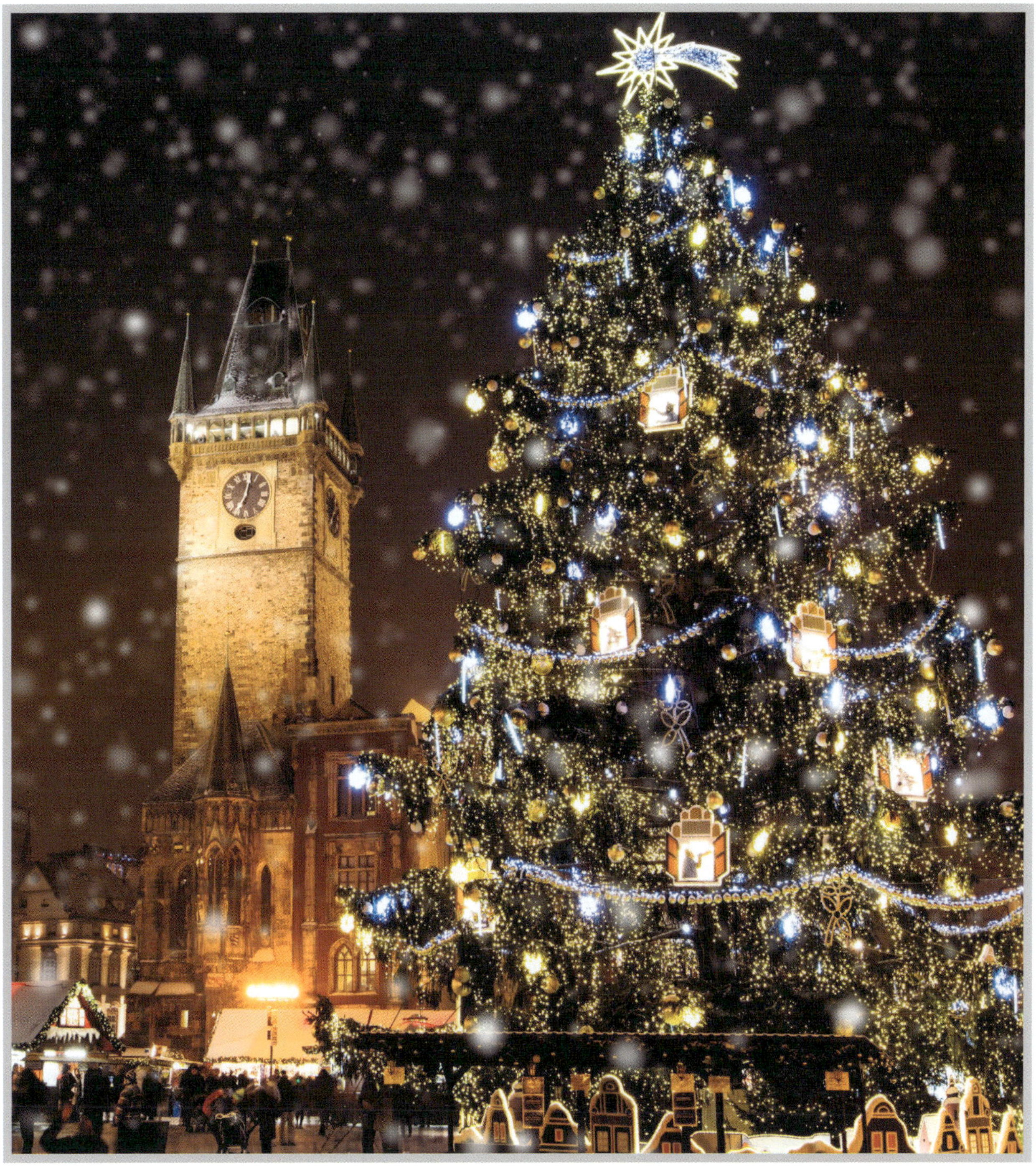

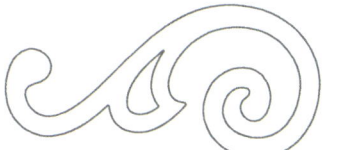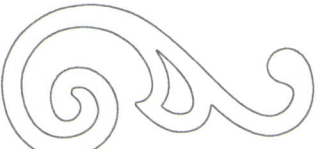

Jingle Bells

Jingle bells, jingle bells,

Jingle all the way.

Oh! what fun it is to ride

In a one-horse open sleigh. Hey!

Jingle bells, jingle bells,

Jingle all the way;

Oh! what fun it is to ride

In a one-horse open sleigh.

James Pierpont

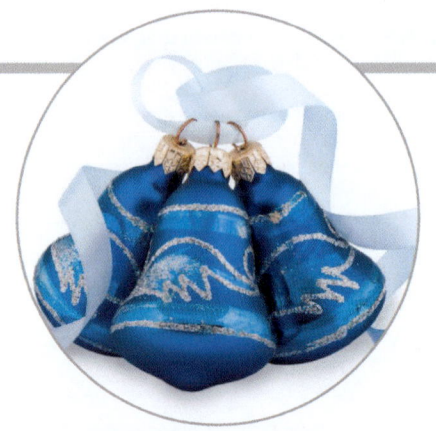

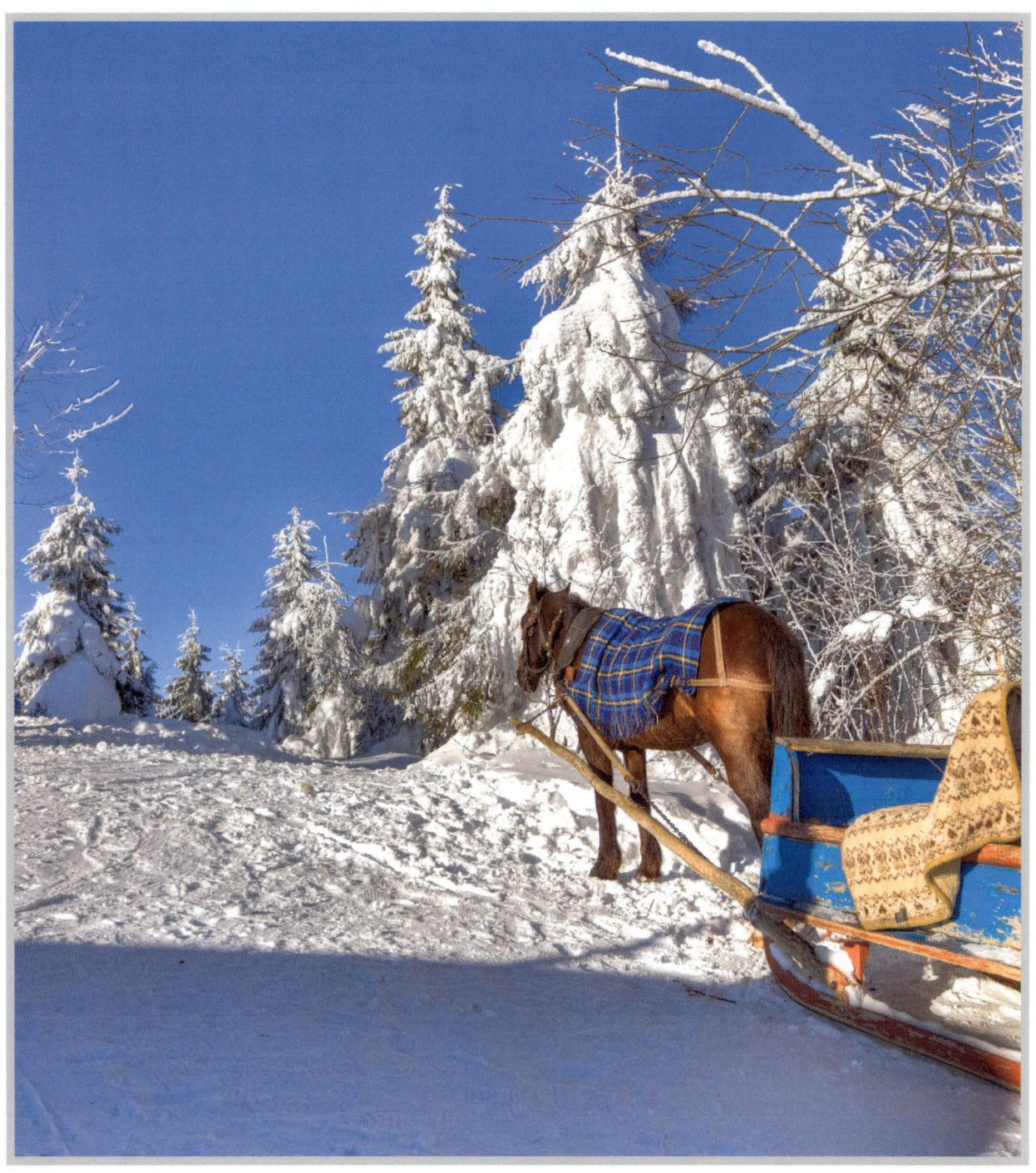

The Night Before Christmas

'Twas the night before Christmas,

when all through the house

Not a creature was stirring,

not even a mouse;

The stockings were hung

by the chimney with care,

In hopes that St. Nicholas

soon would be there.

Clement Clarke Moore

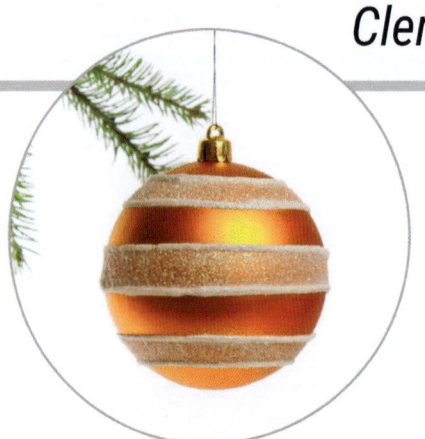

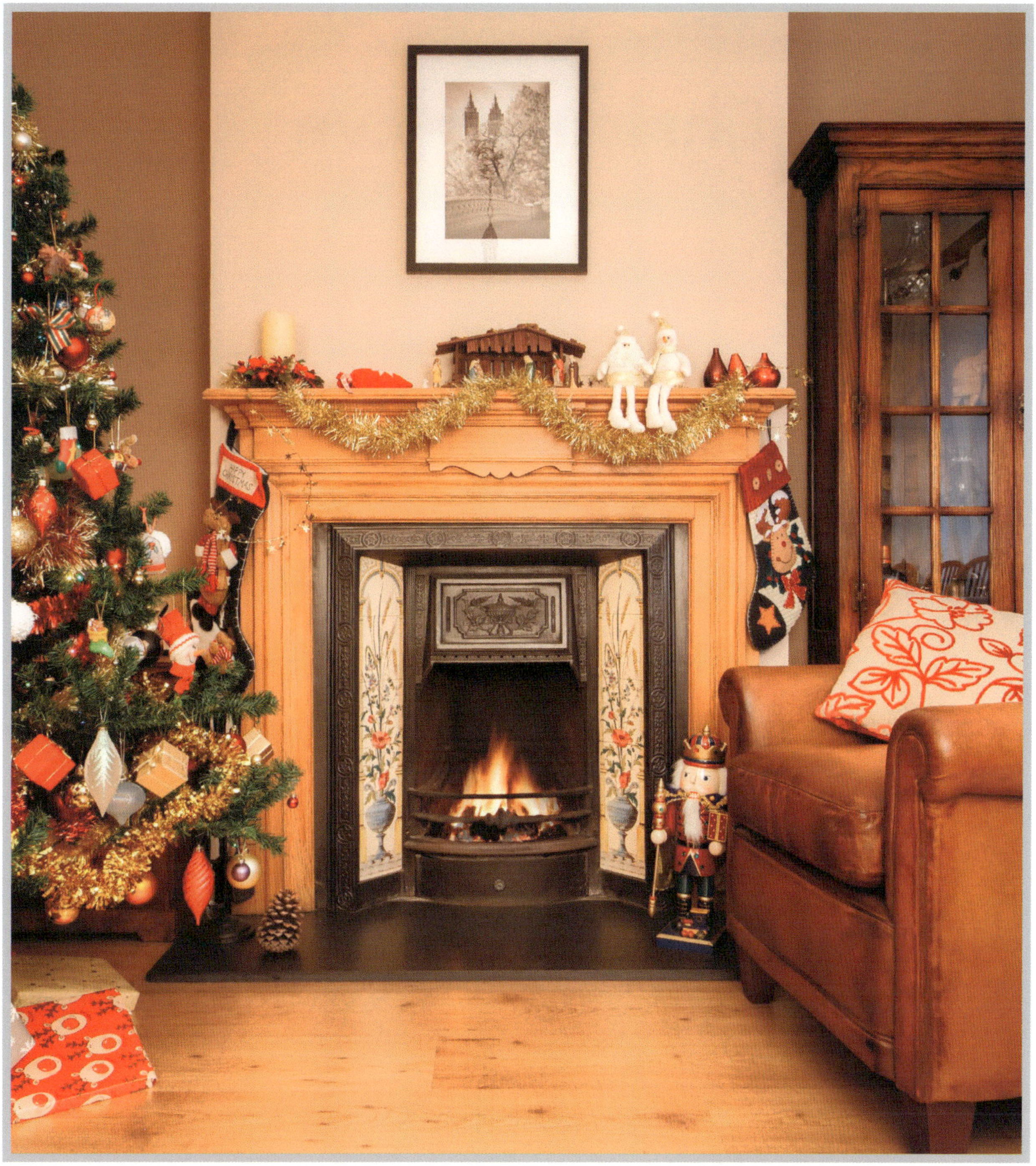

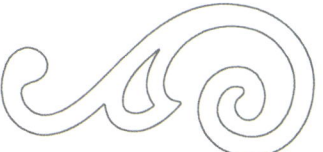
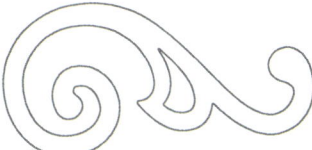

Christmas Eve

Deep lies the snow upon the earth,

But all the sky is ringing

With joyous song, and all night long

The stars shall dance, with singing.

Eugene Field

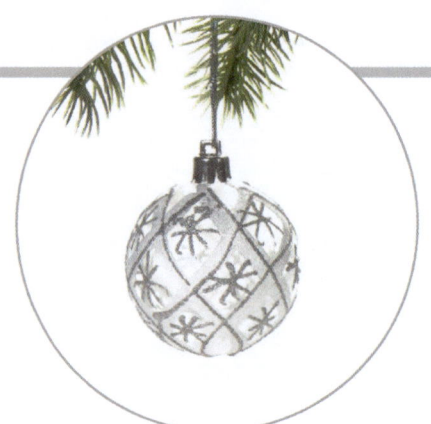

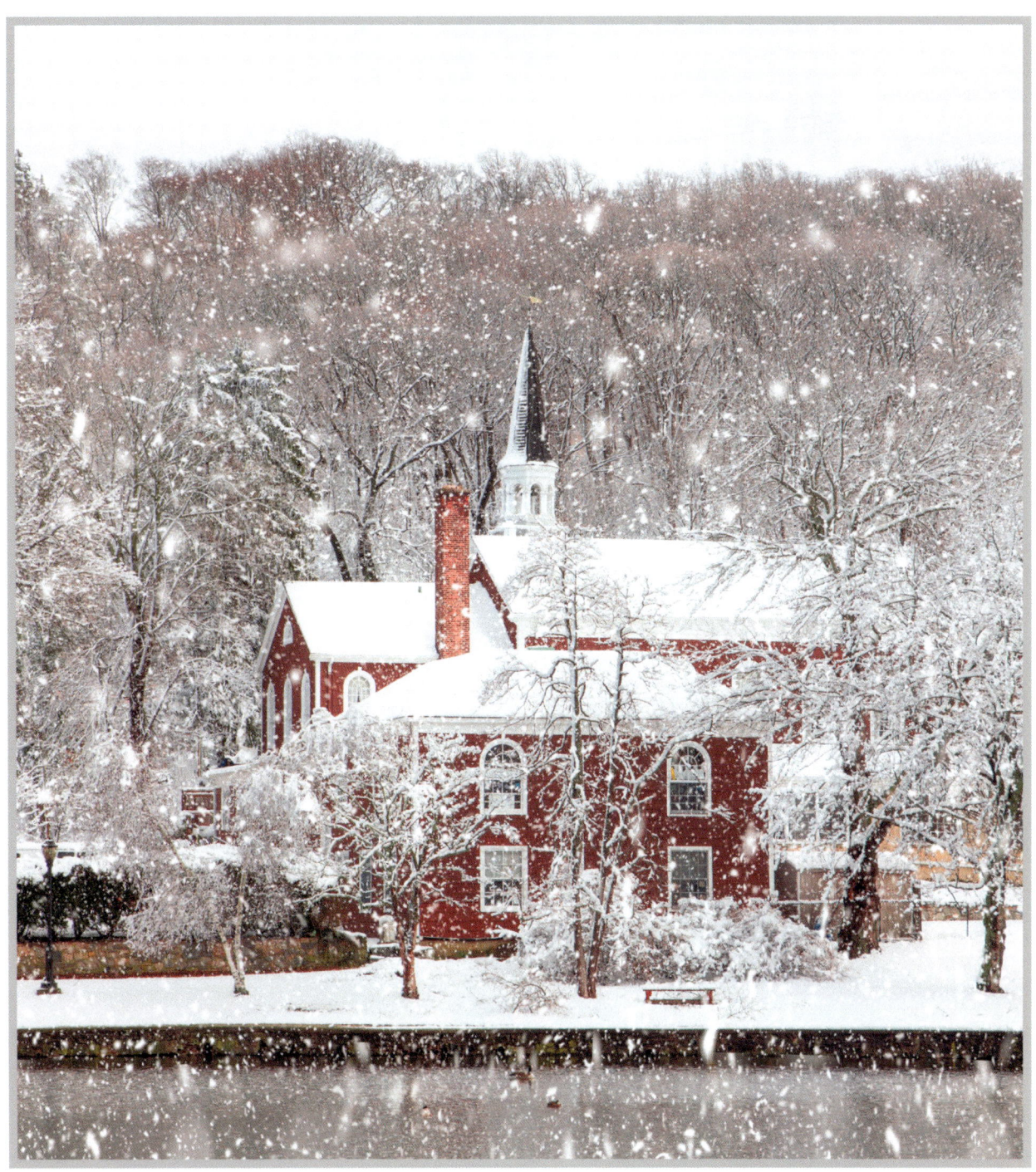

Lordings, Listen to our Lay

Lordings, listen to our lay—

We have come from far away

To seek Christmas;

In this mansion we are told

He His yearly feast doth hold:

'Tis to-day!

May joy come from God above,

To all those who Christmas love.

Traditional carol

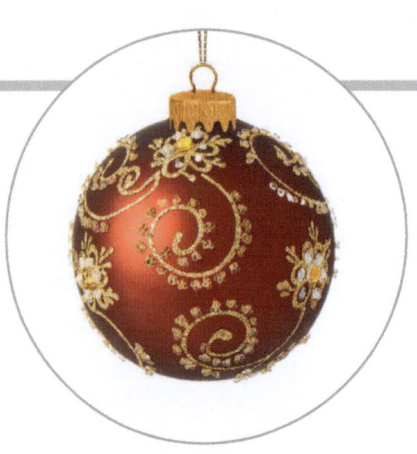

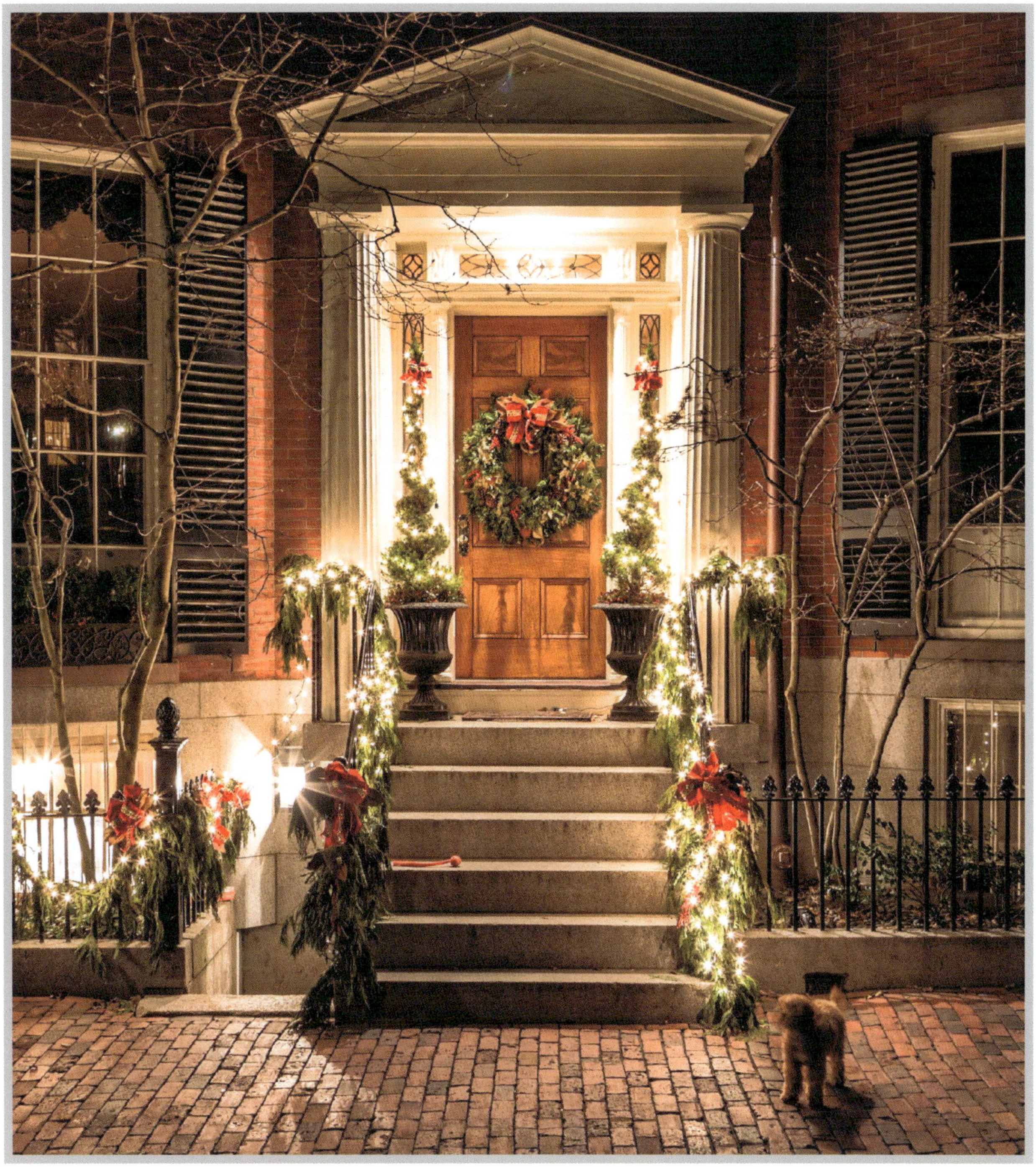

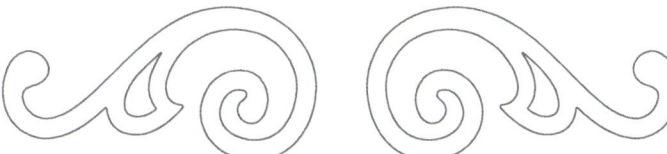

Carol of the Field-Mice

Villagers all, this frosty tide,

Let your doors swing open wide,

Though wind may follow, and snow beside,

Yet draw us in by your fire to bide;

      Joy shall be yours in the morning!

From 'The Wind in the Willows'
Kenneth Grahame

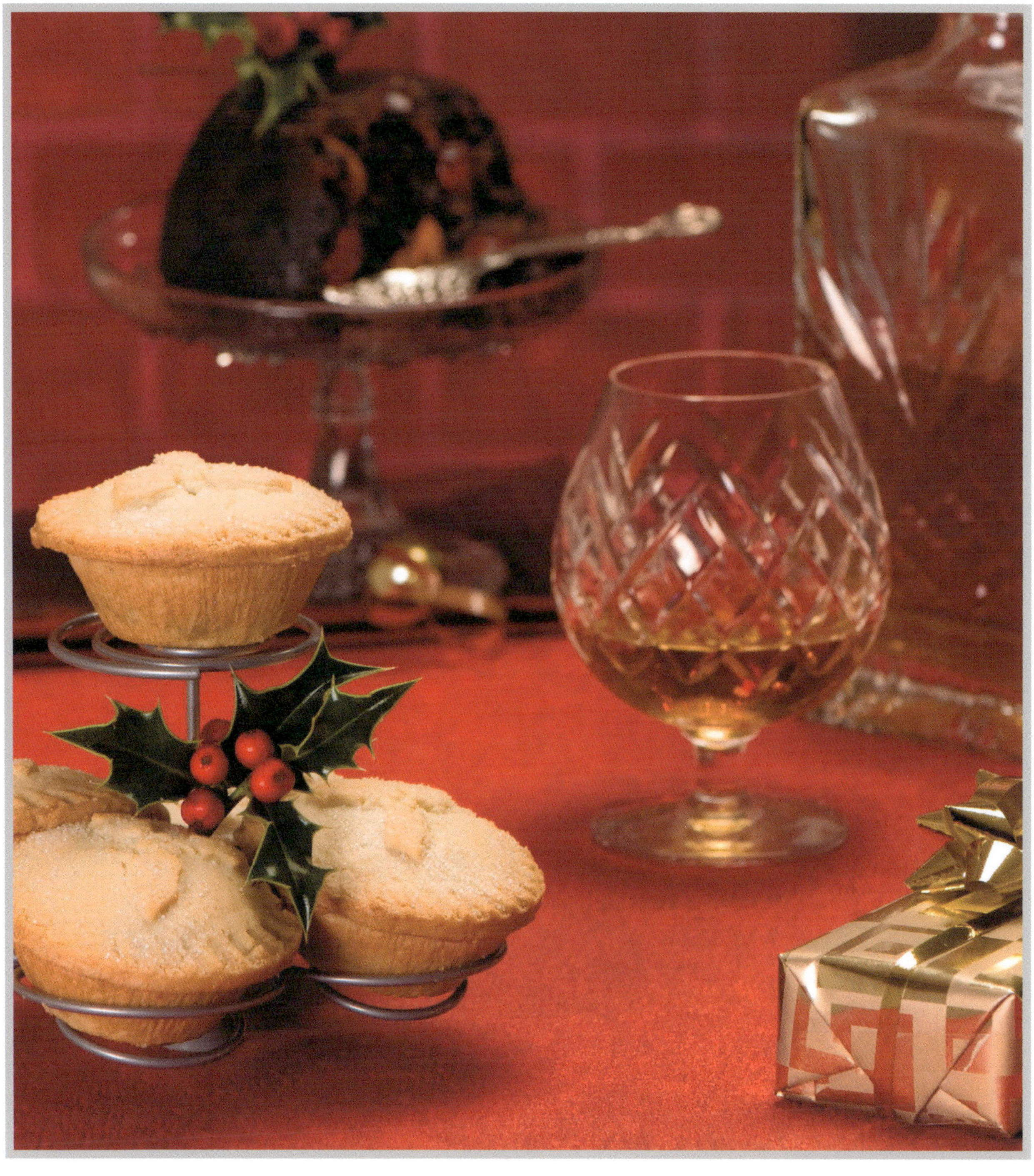

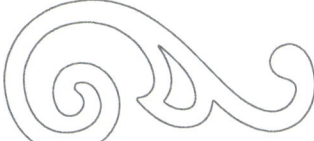

Christmas Morning

Come all you weary wanderers,

Beneath the wintry sky;

This day forget your worldly cares,

And lay your sorrows by;

Awake, and sing

The church bells ring;

For this is Christmas morning!

Edwin Waugh

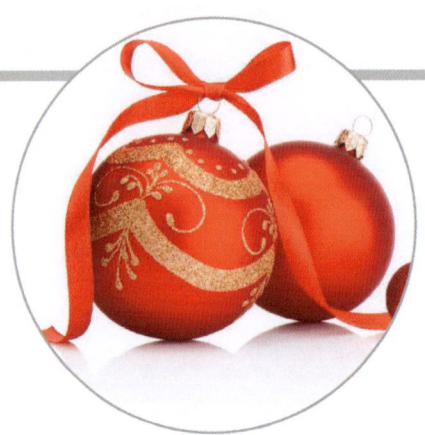

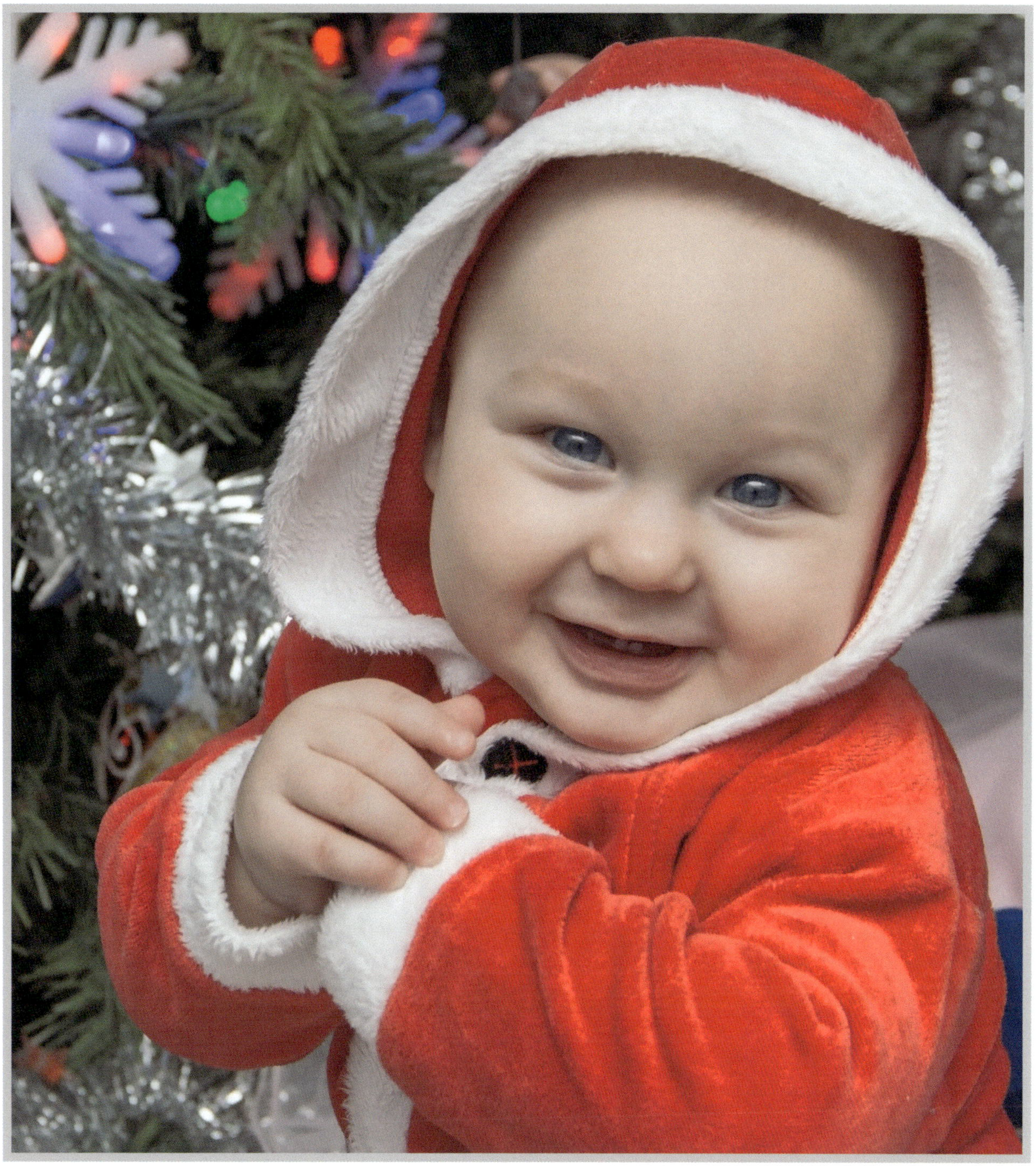

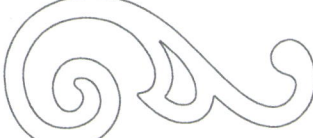

A Christmas Carol

Before the paling of the stars,

Before the winter morn,

Before the earliest cockcrow

Jesus Christ was born:

Born in a stable,

Cradled in a manger,

In the world His hands had made

Born a stranger.

Christina Rossetti

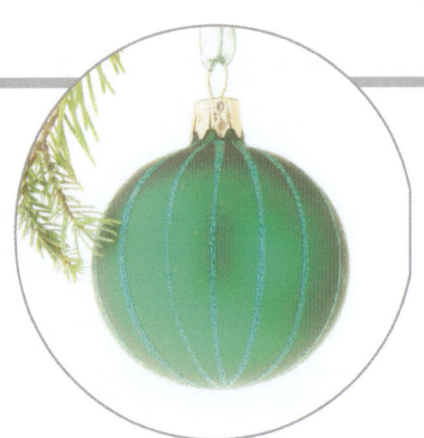

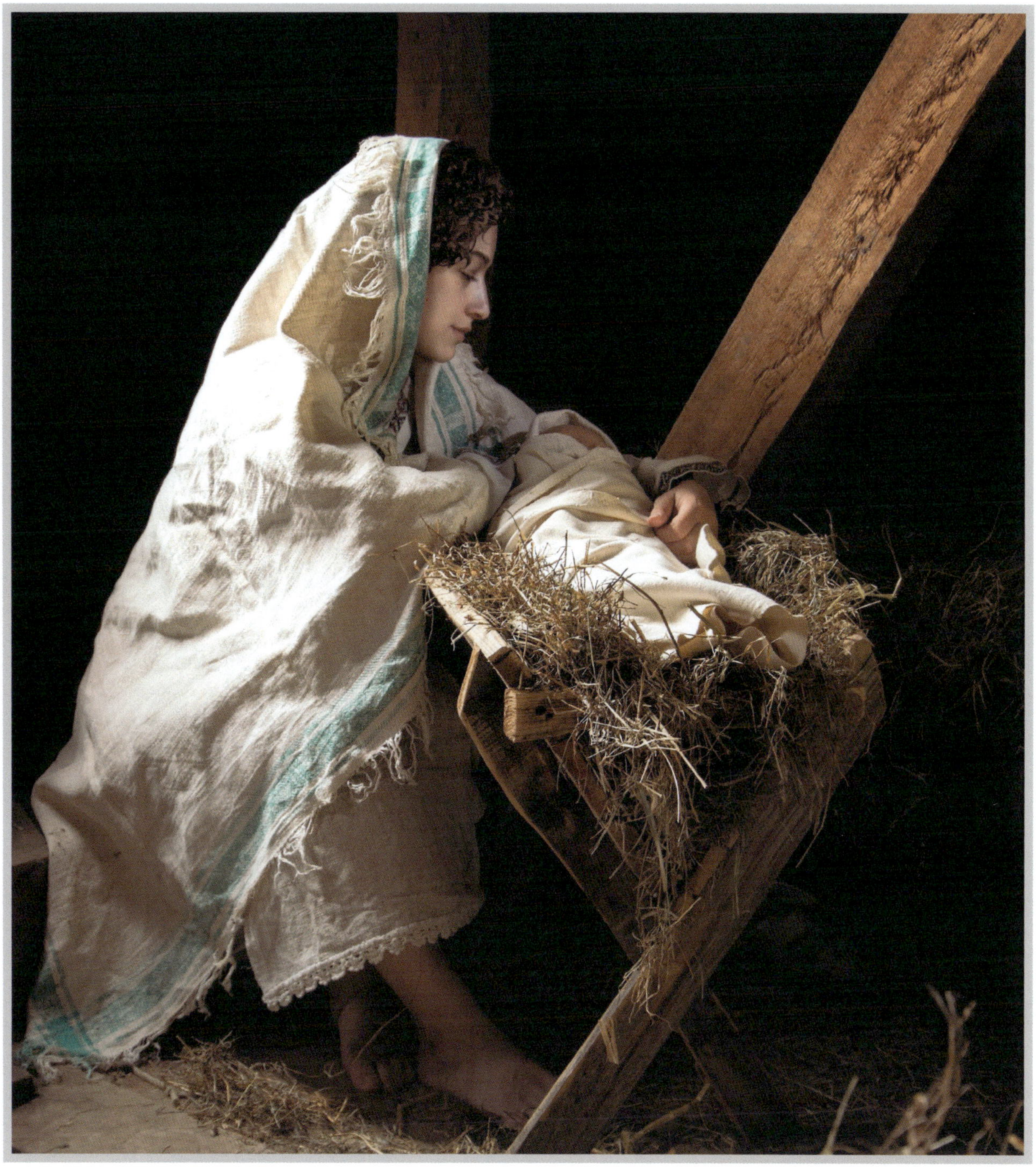

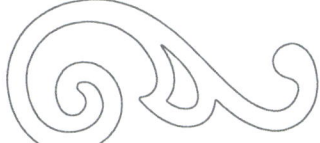

Christmas Bells

I heard the bells on Christmas Day

Their old, familiar carols play,

And wild and sweet the words repeat

Of peace on Earth, good-will to men!

Henry W. Longfellow

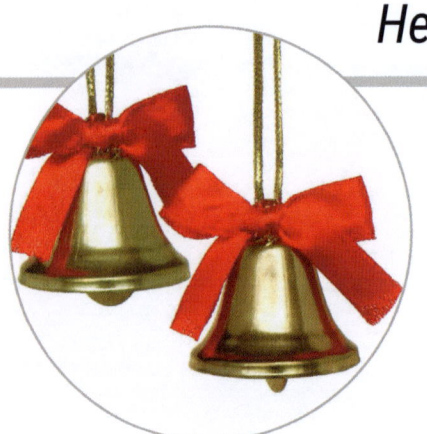

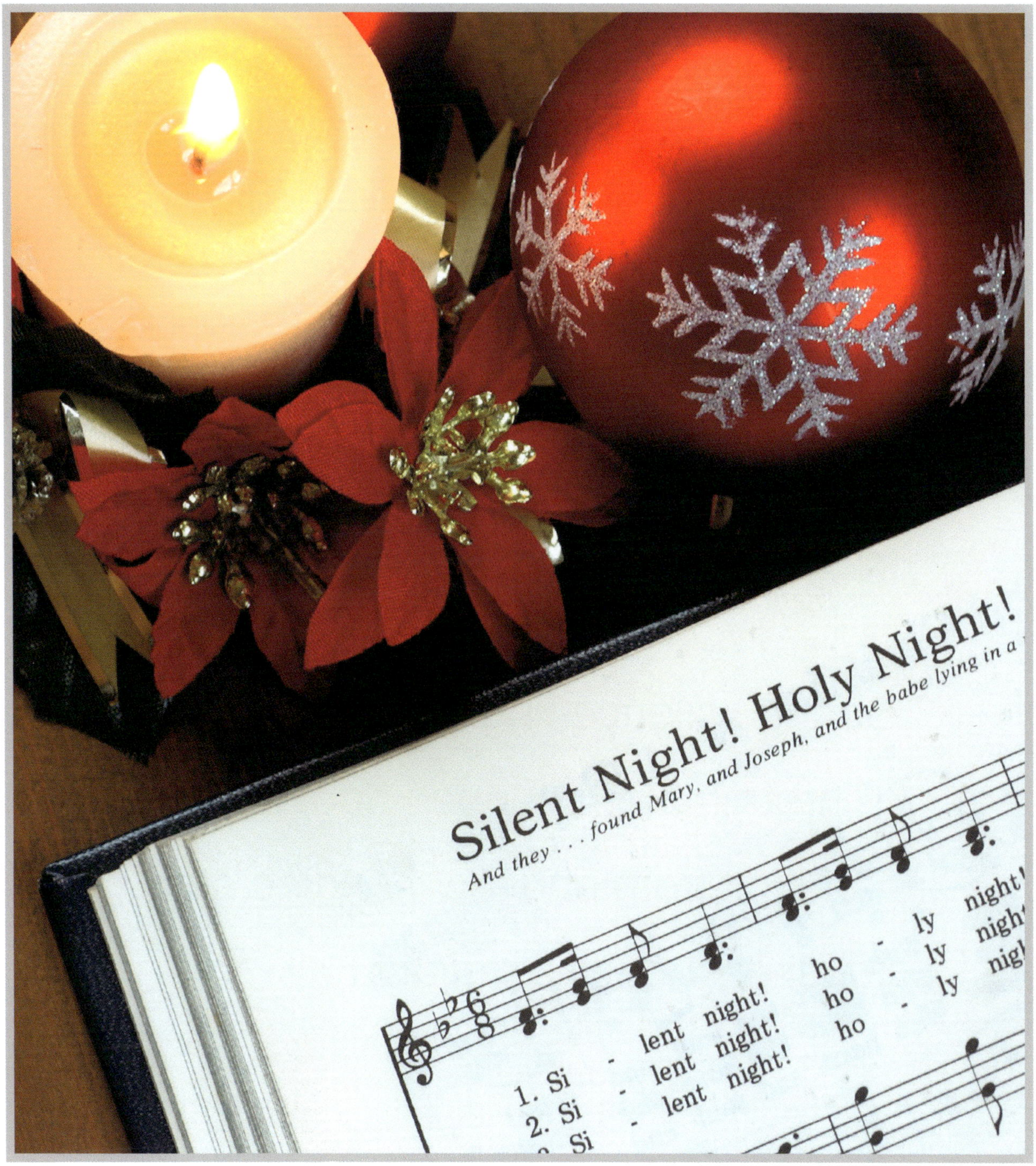

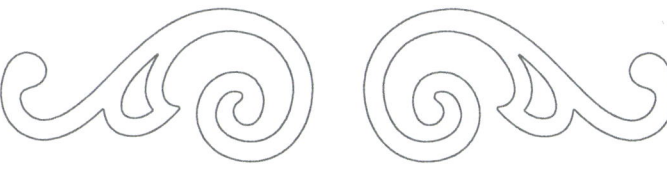

The Christmas Silence

Hushed are the pigeons cooing low
  On dusty rafters of the loft;
  And mild-eyed oxen, breathing soft,
Sleep on the fragrant hay below.

Strange silence tingles in the air;
  Through the half-open door a bar
  Of light from one low-hanging star
Touches a baby's radiant hair.

Margaret Deland

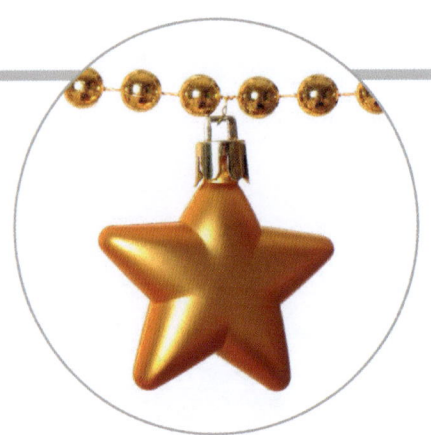

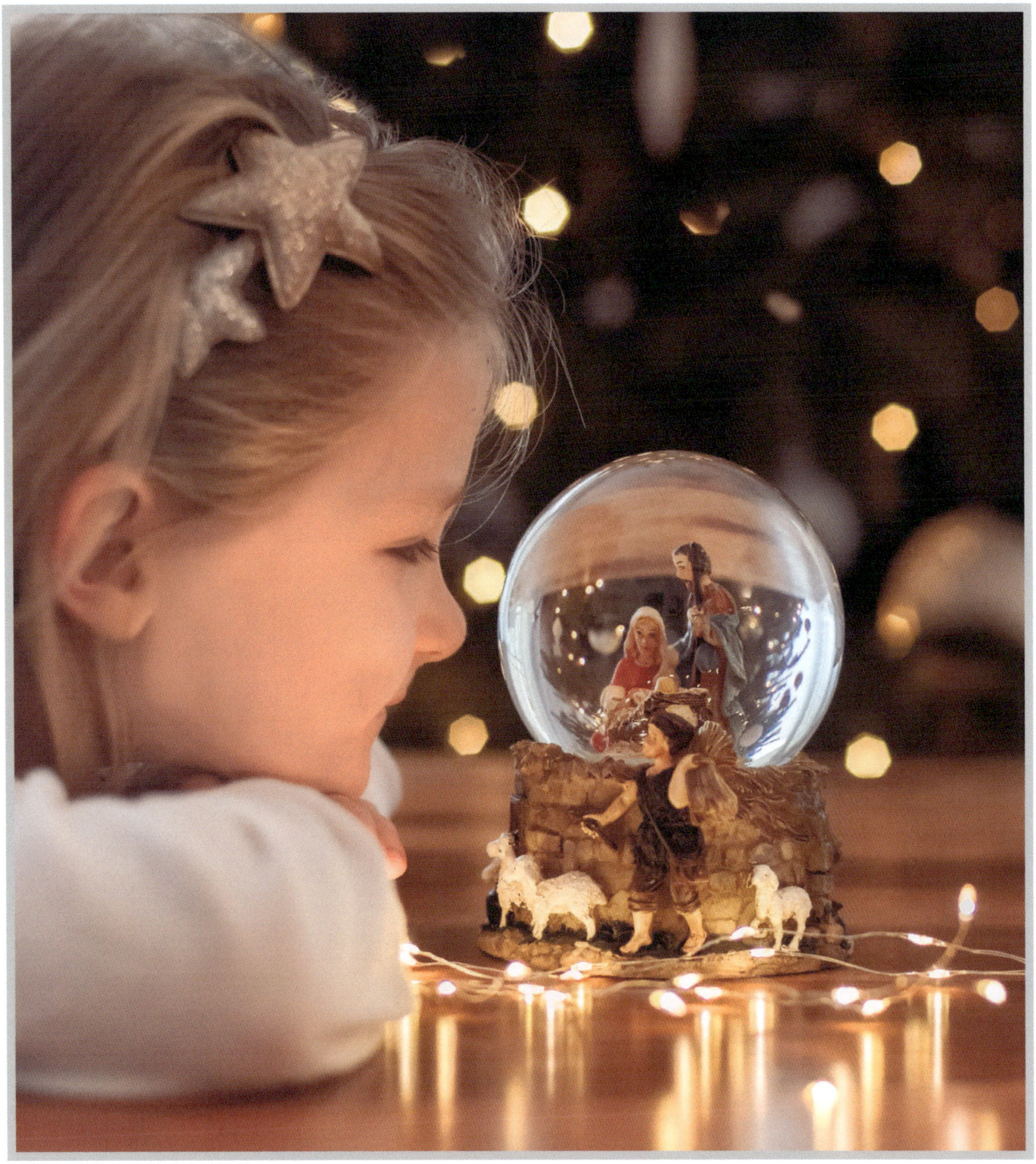

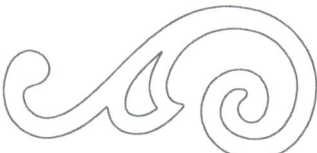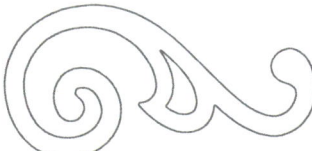

A Christmas Carol

The Christ-child lay on Mary's lap,

His hair was like a light.

(O weary, weary were the world,

But here is all aright.)

The Christ-child stood on Mary's knee,

His hair was like a crown,

And all the flowers looked up at Him,

And all the stars looked down.

G. K. Chesterton

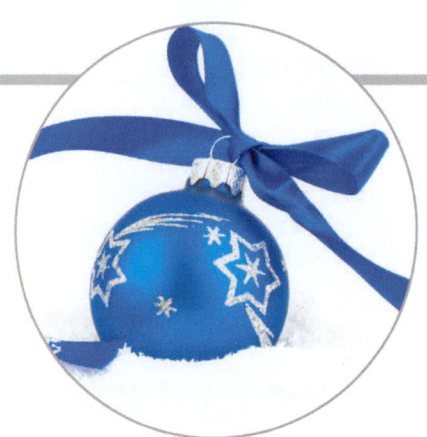

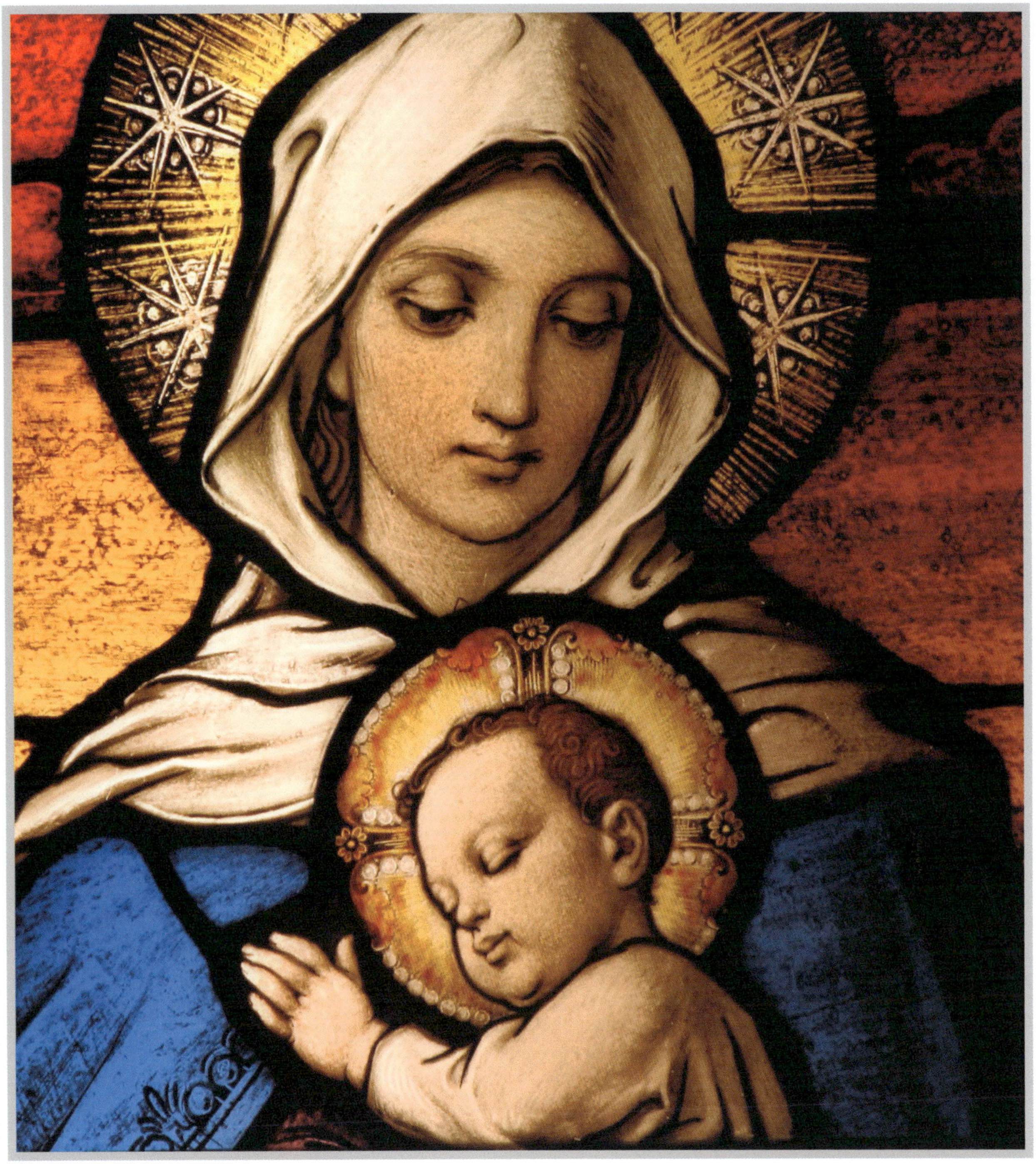

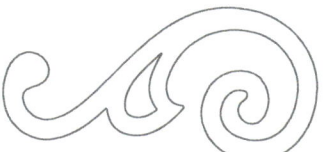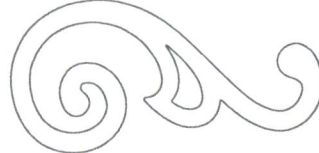

Song for a Christmas Tree

Cold and wintry is the sky,

Bitter winds go whistling by,

Orchard boughs are bare and dry,

Yet here stands a faithful tree.

Household fairies kind and dear,

With loving magic none need fear,

Bade it rise and blossom here,

Little friends, for you and me.

Louisa May Alcott

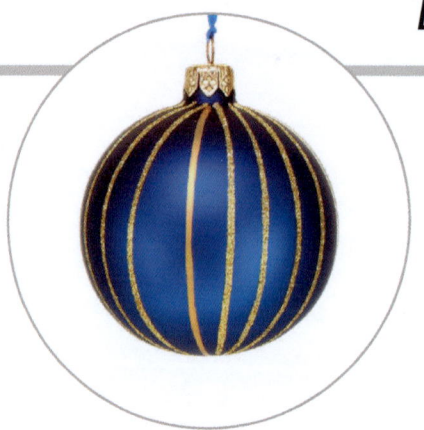

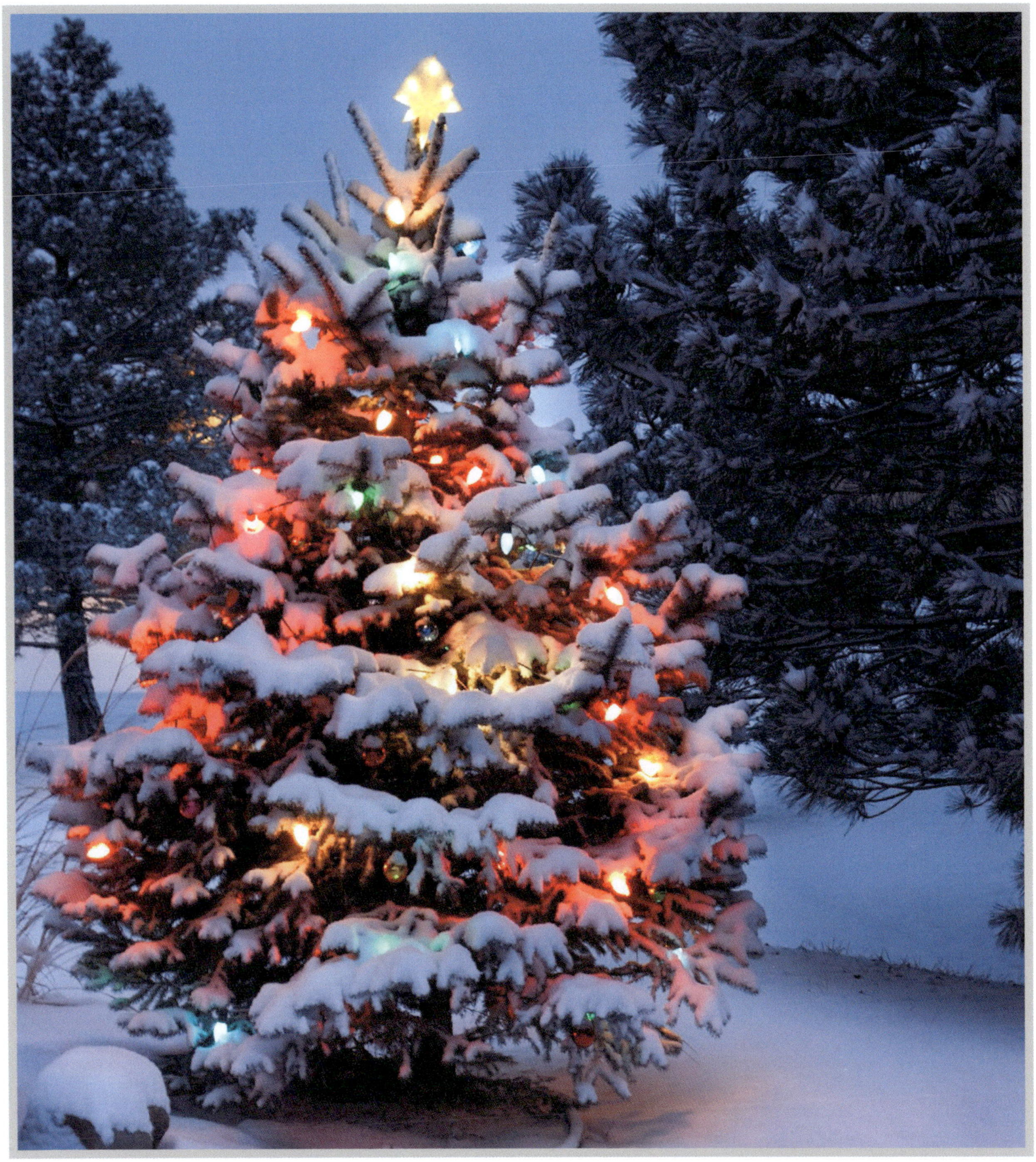

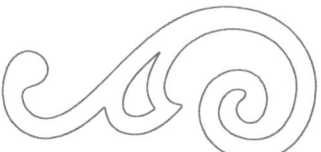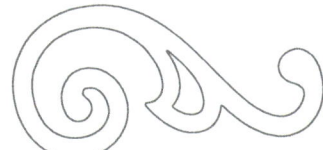

We Wish You a Merry Christmas

We wish you a merry Christmas

We wish you a merry Christmas

We wish you a merry Christmas

   and a happy new year!

Good tidings we bring

   to you and your kin,

We wish you a merry Christmas

   and a happy new year!

Traditional carol

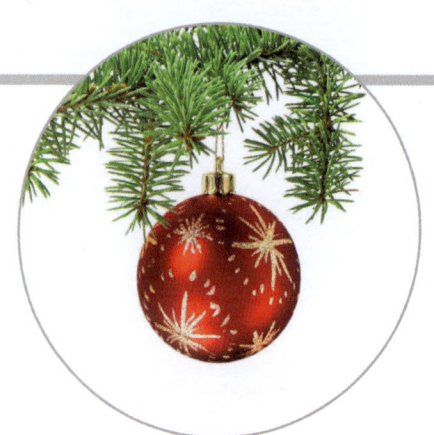

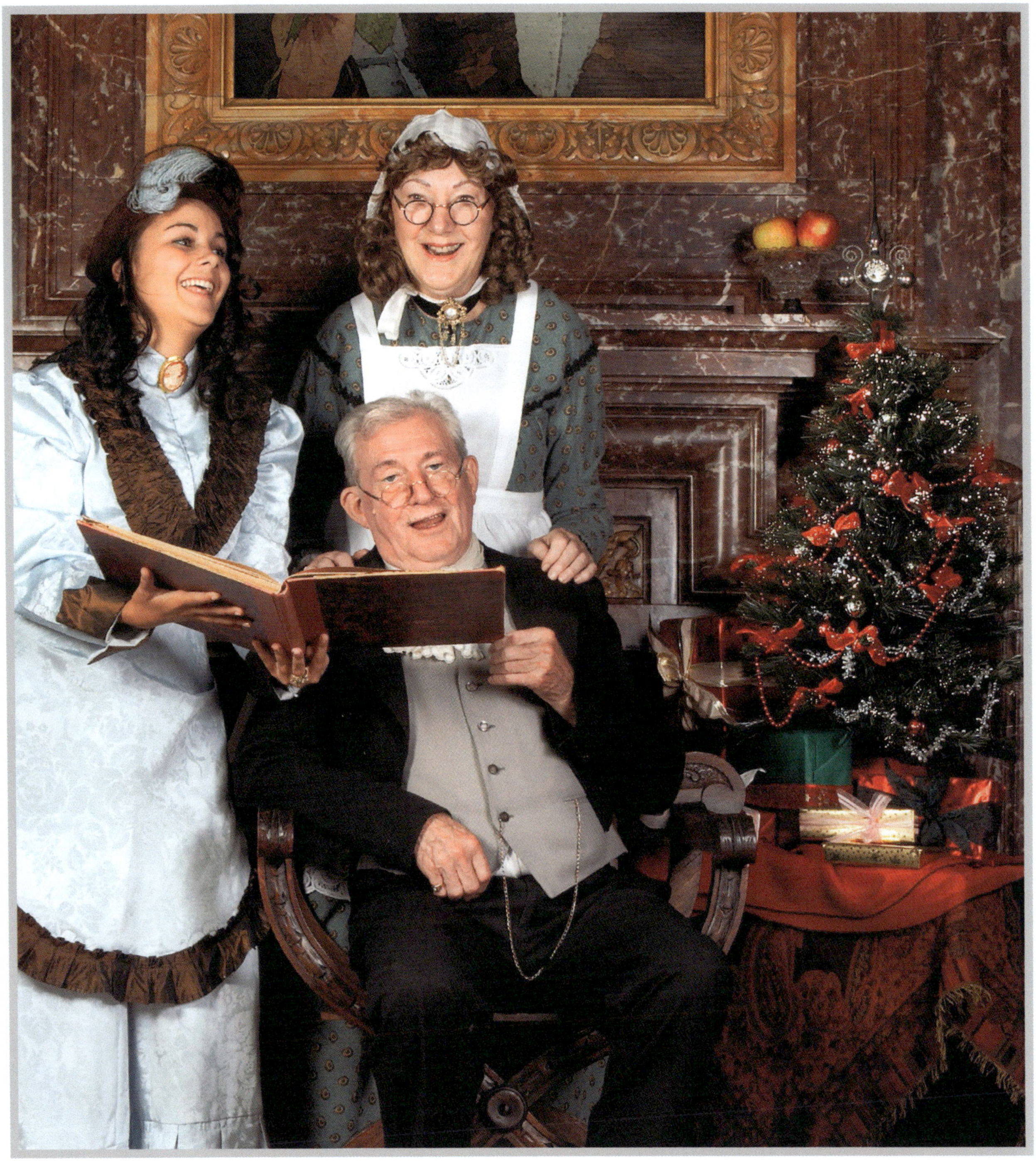

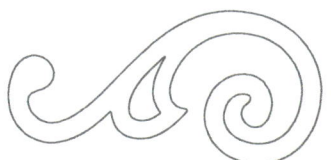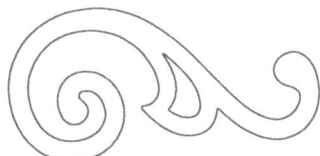

The Christmas Long Ago

Come, sing a hale Heigh-ho

For the Christmas long ago!–

When the old log-cabin homed us

From the night of blinding snow,

Where the rarest joy held reign,

And the chimney roared amain,

With the firelight like a beacon

Through the frosty window-pane.

James Whitcomb Riley

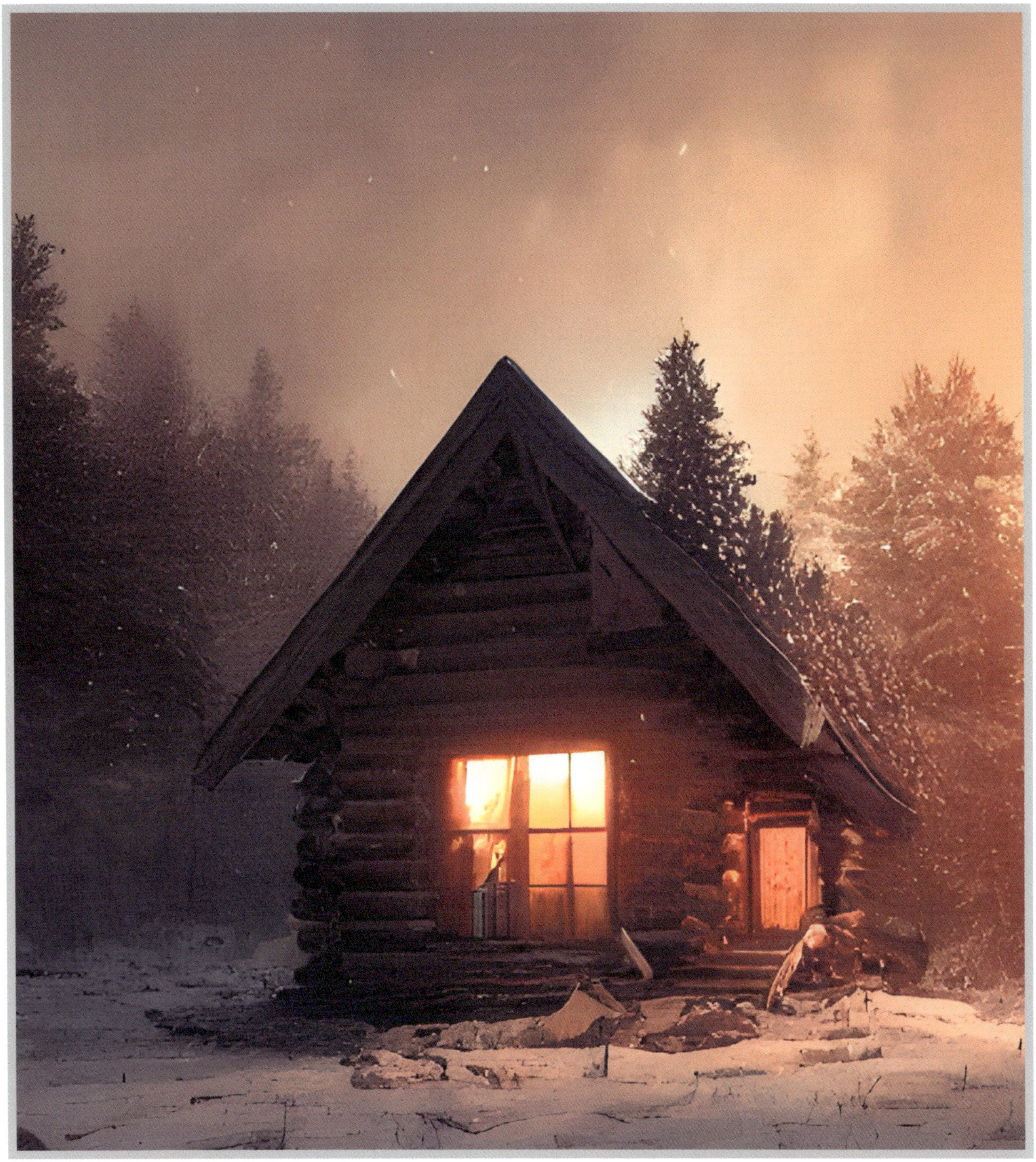

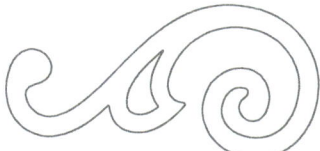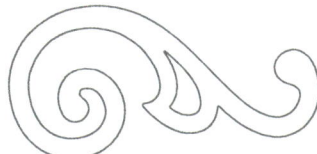

A Yule-Tide Song

Now Christmas is come,

Let us beat up the drum,

And call all our neighbours together,

And when they appear,

Let us make them good cheer,

As will keep out the wind and the weather.

Washington Irving

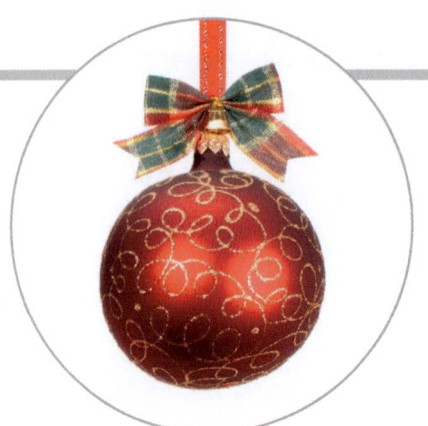

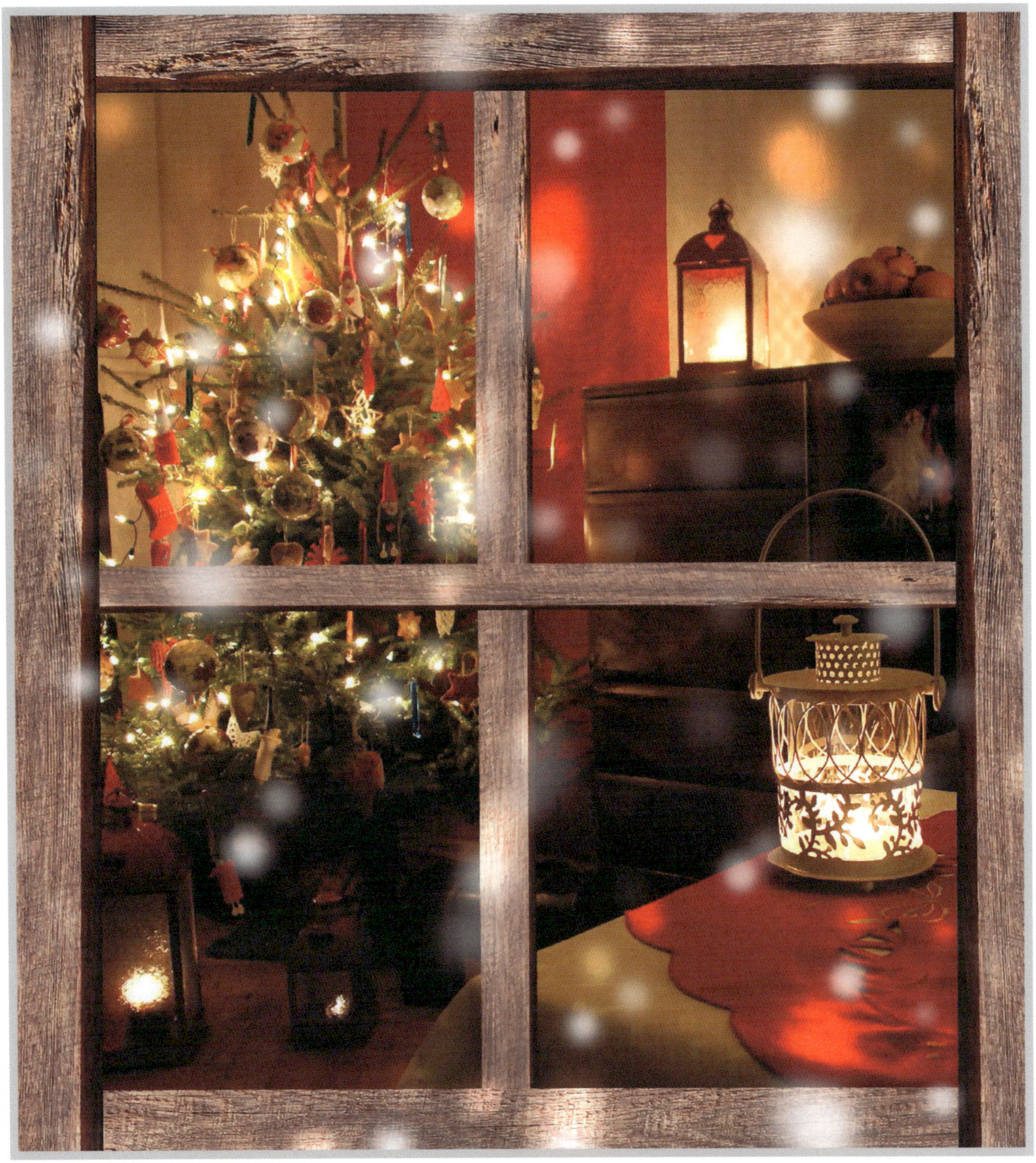

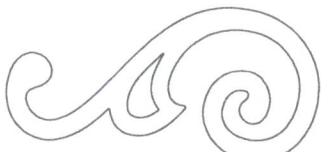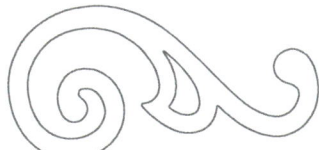

Marmion:
A Christmas Poem

Heap on the wood!

The wind is chill;

But let it whistle as it will,

We'll keep our Christmas merry still.

Sir Walter Scott

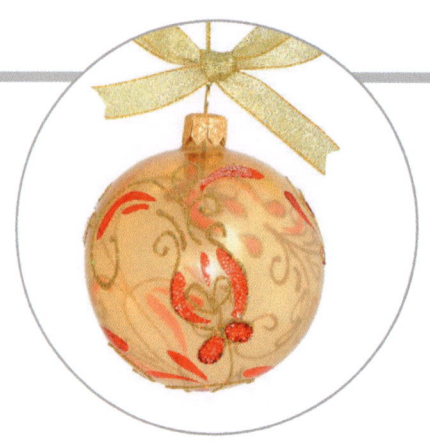

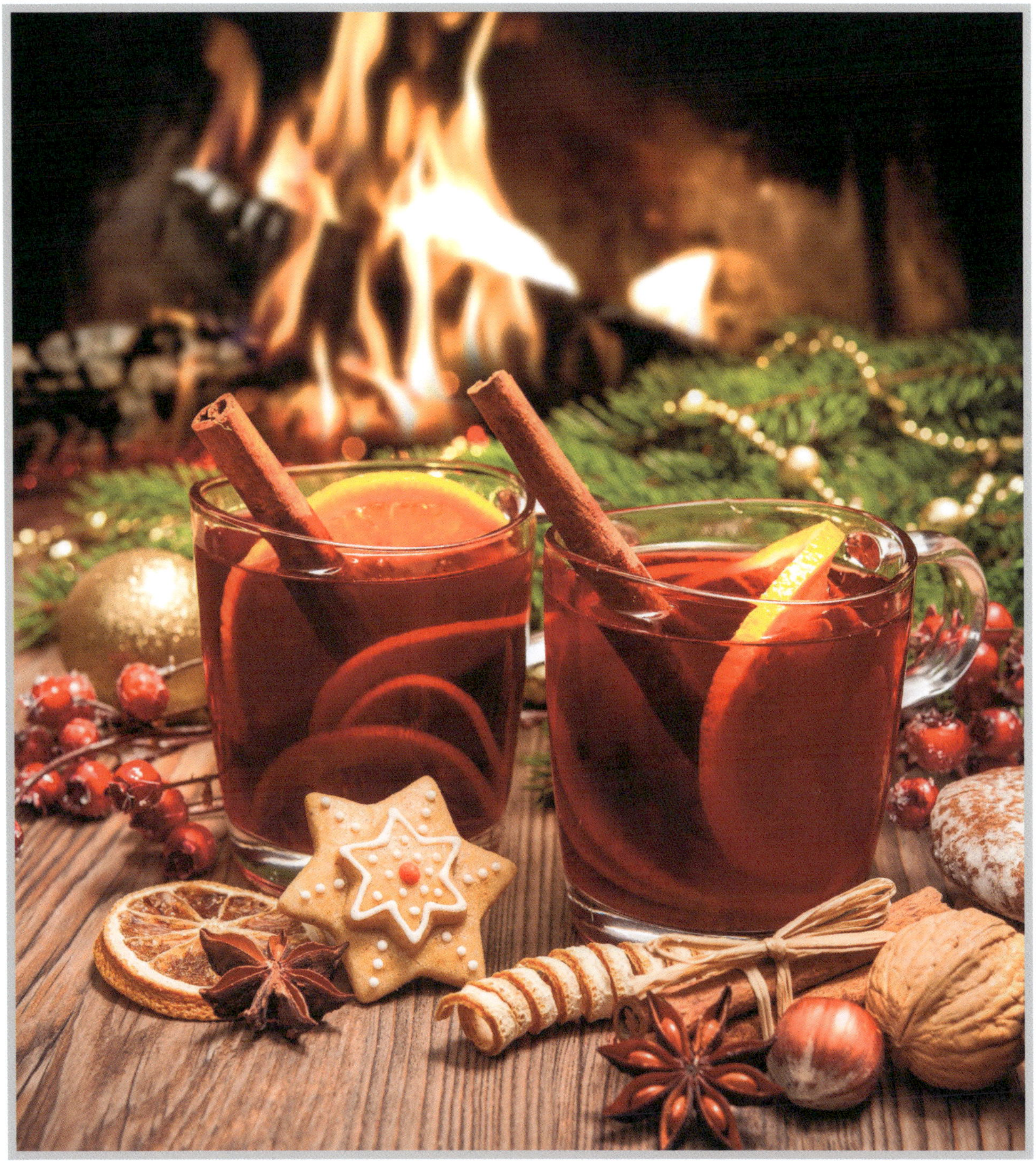

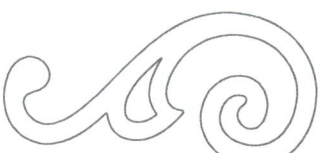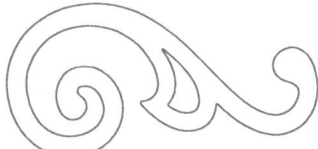

Christmas Sunshine

Do the angels know the blessed day,

And strike their harps anew?

Then may the echo of their lay

Float sweetly down to you,

And fill your soul with Christmas song

That your heart shall echo

your whole life long.

Frances Ridley Havergal

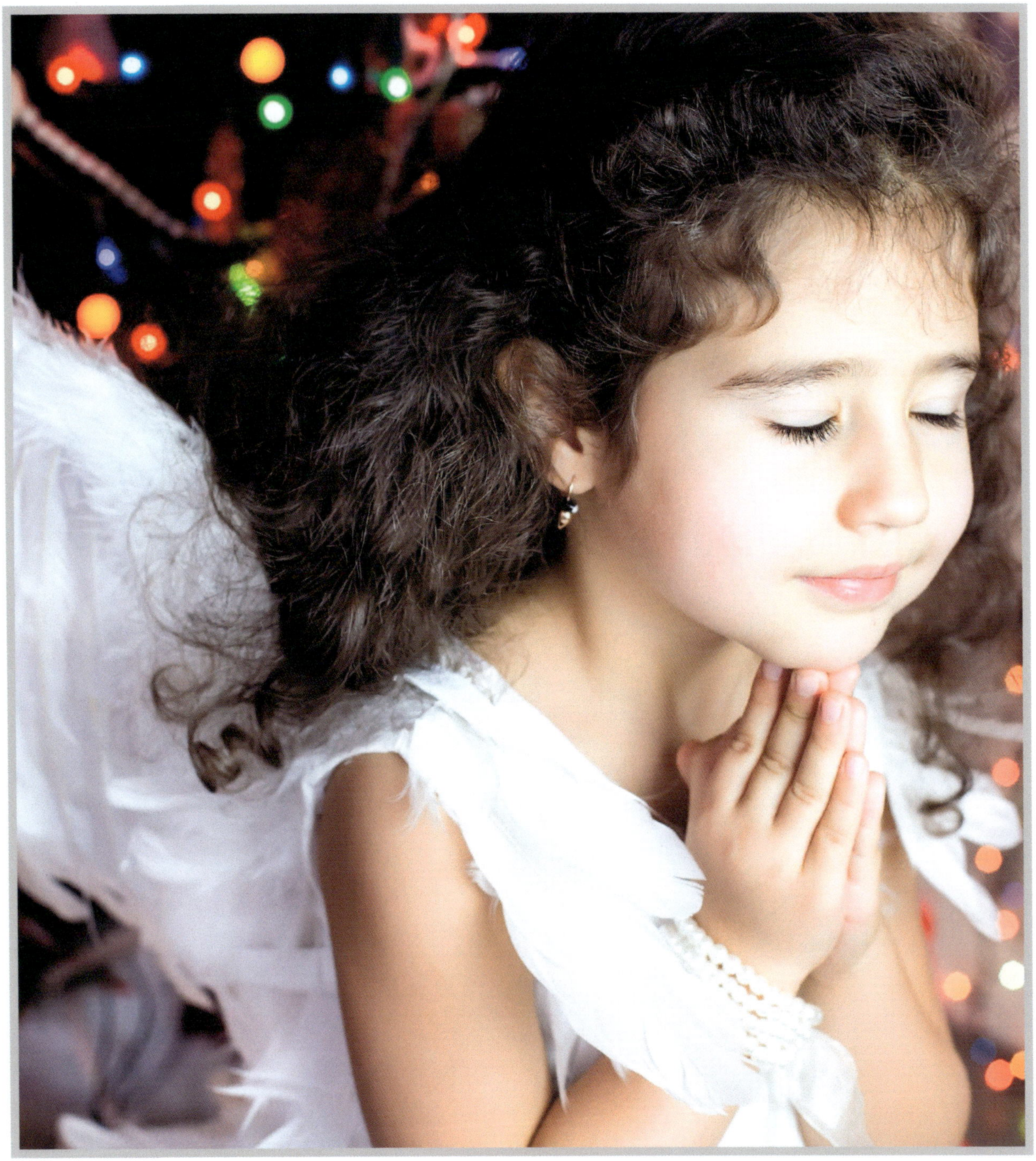

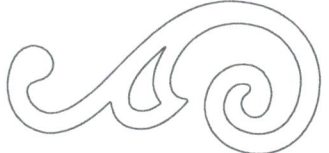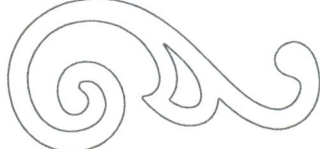

Ring Out, Wild Bells

Ring out the old, ring in the new,

    Ring, happy bells, across the snow:

    The year is going, let him go;

Ring out the false, ring in the true.

Ring in the valiant man and free,

    The larger heart, the kindlier hand;

    Ring out the darkness of the land,

Ring in the Christ that is to be.

Alfred, Lord Tennyson

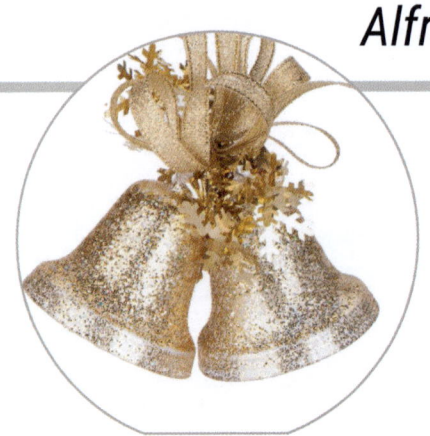

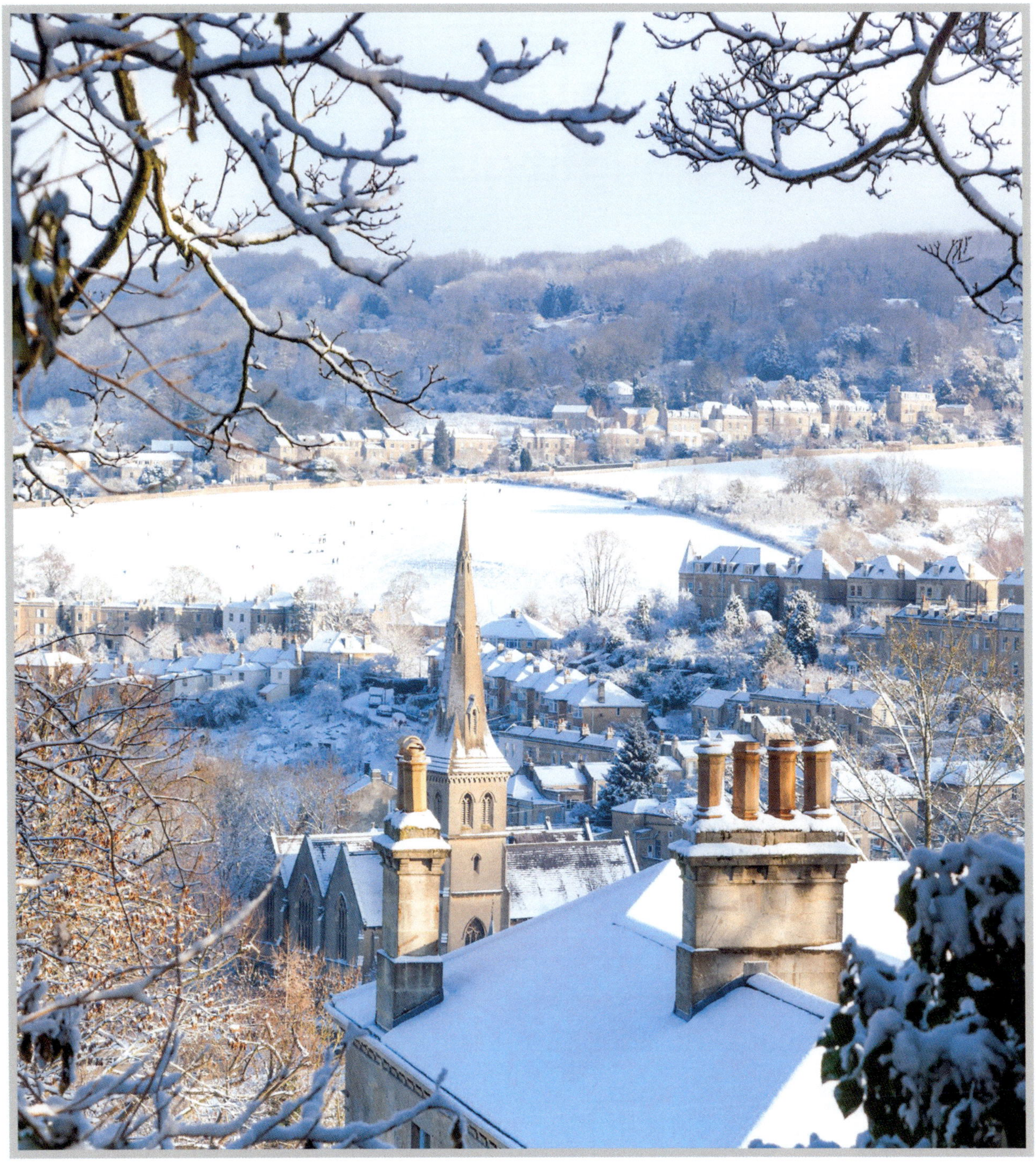

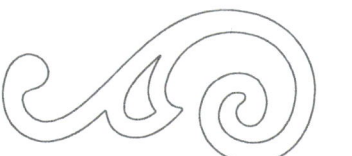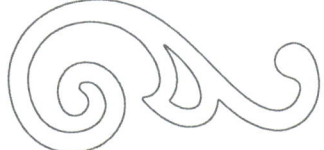

Thank you for reading!
You might also enjoy:

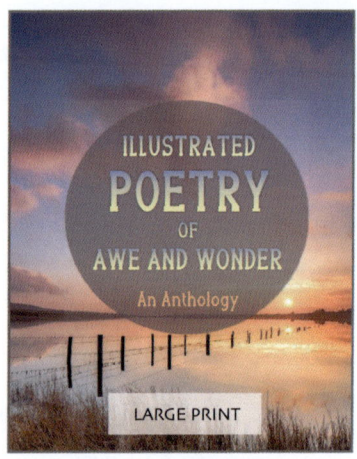

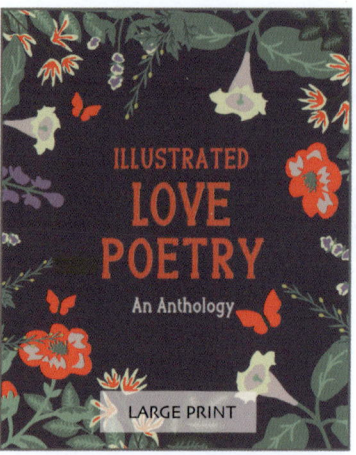

This collection selected by © Unforgettable Notes 2023
All rights reserved. More details at:
thebooknextdoor.com/unforgettablenotes
Huge thanks to Cora de la Cruz (professional advice),
Emma Laybourn (content advice), Jennifer J. Barwick,
Elizabeth Bezant, and the wonderful editing team.
These beautiful poems are in the public domain.

Photos from Deposit Photos: Rfphoto, Hyrman, viktoriya89, eireann, filmfoto, jag_cz, irogova,
maximus19, mr_Brightside, paulmaguire, epitavy, littleny, goir, letf.luis, elnur_, springfield,
Hyrman, PPicasso, griffin024, Marinka, igorot, MKucova, paleka, kipgodi, tinnko,
curaphotography, rojoimages, rcreitmeyer, anterovium, Klanneke, viktoriya89,
ecrafts, Mikha, alga38, a_taiga, alexraths, Hyrman, Mariya_Masich, karandaev, antb

Printed in Great Britain
by Amazon

53657273R00025